Acknowledgements:

I want to thank my Creator, my family, and friends. You all believed in me more than I believed in myself. Thank You Living Foods Institute for your help my walk to the path of freedom.

Forward

This year I chose to live. I started my journey to the rebirth of my mind, body and spirit. I am not finished with my journey. However, if I don't write it down, I will forget and can't share. The journey is not easy as 1, 2, 3 but, it had to be done. And, I am determined to fulfill my promise to my mind, body and spirit to make up for the abuse and neglect. This 10 day cleanse is very liberating. Some steps I will continue to practice and the others performing twice a year.

Introduction

Thank you for purchasing and reading my book. I hope you get just as much from this book as I have. There is nothing new under the sun. With that being said, my book is made up of research I have done of people smarter than me.

Many people ask me "Cissy where do I start? What do I eat? I need help!" Well here it is! This is just the beginning of your walk. We can talk again on where to go next.

Before you start, I want to say a couple of things:

1. Please consult your Doctor. Some things are not for you and your diet.
2. Please watch the video link provided on the liver cleanse.
3. Prepare your foods ahead of time, so you won't get burned out.
4. You may adjust the recipes, just don't leave anything out.
5. Use as many organic products as possible.
6. Remember our journey will not be the same.
7. Keep a journal.
8. Please make your dressings
9. You may have to take baby steps to get through the entire 10 days.

Before you try cleansing, please consult your physician.

Table of Content

Why do I need to Cleanse?

I believe in cleansing your mind, body, and spirit. If your oil in your car is dirty, it affects the engine. You won't get the gas mileage you want out of your car. If the air filters are dirty, it also affects the performance of the car. It is the same with your body. If your colon is not clean, it releases toxins in our body. You eventually smell it in your breath and sometimes through your skin. Cleansing your organs and eating healthy will give you energy; help you to lose the toxic weight and thinking. I believe in cleaning all six areas of your being.

What Type of Cleanse do I need?

1. Spirit
2. Skin
3. Lungs
4. Kidney
5. Liver
6. Colon

Spiritual Cleanse

10 days

The spiritual cleanse was and still is the hardest of all 6 cleanses I have done. Many of us don't want to face ourselves or the truth. We hold onto the past and the pain. Not only do we hold on to it, we nurture it. It becomes a person. My interpretation of the movie "Beloved" is that the mom held onto her past and pain until it manifested into a person. It took over her life. She finally said enough of this. Success, failure, bondage and freedom is in the mind. I had to do this. Freeing yourself for these 10 days is no party. However, it is worth every painful moment. The tears will flow like a river of life restoring your soul. You should experience true freedom. I conquered me.

Meditation, prayer, affirmations, faith, belief and action is the process.

First you must acknowledge the one that gives you breath. I am not all knowing, so I will not say who the I am, but he is. So feed into your source. Someone said there are as many ways to the Creator as there are people. Well said. After you realize that spiritual healing and cleansing does not come from you and you need the help of our Creator (that is whoever the creator puts in your path also), you are ready for the rest.

I believe in prayer talking to your creator. You tell him your concerns and your fears. You ask for help for you and anyone else. This is personal. There are no set words for this. They are the words you choose. He understands them all. In our religious services, we sometimes use elaborate words, but, when we are in need right now, it is "Hey! I need Help!!"

Meditation to me is being still and listening to your creator, your body, and your intuition. I try to meditate twice a day. It gives you peace and clarity. With meditation, I incorporate breathing exercises. There are many meditation techniques. Research them and find what helps you the most. I don't want to give you a specific one because what works for me may not work for you.

Affirmations are the best. It is boosting yourself up and speaking into the universe (Declaring, Claiming it) what you want to come back to you. "I am healed. I will make a change. I release the toxins. I welcome the good." Saying them and believing them will bring your desires back to you.

Now, put it all into action. Walk and act like it is already happening. This is your victory walk. You have to make things happen.

I truly believe the spirit must take control of every situation and make it work. If you don't believe, it will not happen. If you can't see it, it won't happen.

So make it happen!!!

Skin Cleanse:

10 days

The skin is the largest organ of the body. Just like the others it must be cleaned and exercised. It is said that rosemary and vitamin e is great for the skin. I actually make body butter with both ingredients in it and it feels wonderful. I do feel the difference. There are a several ways to detox your skin. The ones I tried are skin brushing, water intake, and sweating it out.

Skin brushing is good for your lymphatic system, your circulation, exfoliation, and overall appearance.
Skin brushing is new to me. In an article Dr. Edward explains the technique:

To perform skin brushing, clean your body by taking a shower or bath. Then, making sure your skin is completely dry, gently move the bristles of a natural loofah sponge or boar bristle brush along your skin, using strokes that begin at the heart and slowly move outwards

I believe the easiest for me is drinking plenty of water and sweating it out. Intake of water is important. Water carries out the toxins. Water hydrates your body and is great for the skin. I have pretty decent skin, however when I drink the water required, I get so many compliments on my skin.

You are to drink half of your body weight in ounces daily. Example: 100lbs 50 ounces of water.

Sweat it out, Sweat, Sweat Sweat.
I never thought sweating was too cute. Girls don't sweat. Oh, how wrong I was. When I come out of the sauna or the steam room, I feel wonderful. (Side note: use sauna for 10 or 15 minutes before exercising. It relaxes your muscles) Also, sweating when exercising helps get the toxins out. So, make

sure you get in your water and exercise. For the sake of completely cleansing, it will be done the entire 10 days. This is a cleanse you should do always

Lung Cleanse
10 day process

The Lung cleanse is a simple one but just as important. Most of us don't breathe deep. We are shallow breathers. I believe when you inhale you welcome life and when you exhale you denounce negativity. It also pulls the oxygen into our blood cells and carriers out the carbon dioxide.

Exercise:

Inhale from your noise and fill your belly with as much air as possible.

Hold your breath for 5 seconds and exhale.

Repeat this 6 times. Participate in this process 3 times a day.

Feel the stress leave your body.

Kidney Cleanse
5 days

The kidneys are a major organ in your body and they are responsible for clearing waste from your body. The kidneys also, balance body fluids, from urine, and help in other important functions of the body. Every day the kidneys process the blood to sift out waste products and extra water.

This is a Five day drinking only cleanse. It may be challenging to some. If you need to eat, make sure it is raw vegetables.

Liver and Colon Cleanse

3 days

We know the liver carries good nutrients to the body and the bad away. It also stores glucose. When eating a lot of greasy, fatty and fried foods, the liver accumulates stones. The stones are made cholesterol, lipids (fat), bile pigments, protein, bile salts, biliary sludge and bilirubin. This is what we want to get rid of in this cleanse. You can research in depth what all the organs do in your spare time.

The colon carries waste from your body. It eliminates the things your body doesn't need. You can take care of both of the cleanses at the same time. I don't like pills, so I chose the Dr. Hulda's cleanse without the sleeping pill. It is done with food and epsom salt. It is a 4 day process.

You can get great instructions and the ingredients from 'you tube' for this process at: https://www.youtube.com/watch?v=xXTUVDRkZCA. It is called,"Doing the Hulda Clark Liver Cleanse"

I can tell you from experience I passed about five hundred stones. I can wear perfume now. Before you try this process, please consult your doctor. Some wait 2 weeks and repeat the process.

I hope I have made the 10 day process clear for you. You're probably asking what happens after I go through this process. I'm not going to leave you out on a limb. We will discuss different foods to eat and how to combine your foods in my next book.

It is your choice on which path to walk for your continued freedom. Whether you become a raw foodist, vegan, vegetarian or start choosing healthier foods for your body is up to you. What is required for my mind, body and spirit is not the same as what will make your engine purr. I encourage you to research, try new things, and listen to your body and spirit.

Welcome to freedom!

Day by Day

Day 1

Spirit: (minimum)

Prayer	once daily
Mediation	twice a day

Skin

Brushing	once daily
Water	Drink ½ of your body weight in ounces

daily

Sweat	Daily

Lungs

Deep breathing	all day
Breathing Exercise	3 times a day

Food to eat day 1:

Morning Glory (Daily Shake) Inspired by Living Foods Institute

3 cups of greens
2 cups of seeds (sprouted)
2 cups of sprouts
½ apple
½ avocado
2 tbl sea vegetable (**Chlorella, Dulse, Kelp, Nori** (aka laver), **Spirulina, Wakame)**
sprouted
Himalayan salt (to taste)
Cayenne pepper
                 Drink this smoothie all day if you like.

Salad (Large) Choose from the following Vegetables:

Arugula
Bok choy
Broccoli
Brussels sprouts
Turnips
Cauliflower

Horseradish
Kale
Radishes
Rutabaga
Cabbage
Watercress

Snack

Kale Chips

If you don't have a dehydrator, go to a raw foods restaurant and pick some up. Cut up some Kale sprinkle oil, Himalayan salt, garlic, nutritional yeast. Place in the dehydrator on 105 for 4 hours. If they are not as crispy as you like, dehydrate until you are satisfied.

Raw Popcorn

1 head of cauliflower, onion powder, garlic powder Himalayan salt olive oil. Cut up the Cauliflower, and add all the ingredients to taste. You may add other spices you like. You can place in the dehydrator for 30 minutes or eat without dehydrating.

Raw veggie packs

Cut up your choice of veggies from above and put in baggies to carry around all day.

Day 2 - 6

Spirit: (minimum)

Prayer	once daily	
Mediation	twice a day	

Skin

Brushing	once daily	
Water	Drink ½ of your body weight in ounces

daily

Sweat	Daily

Lungs

Deep breathing	all day
Breathing Exercise	3 times a day

Kidney Cleanse
Day 2-4 Drink: Morning Glory, Drink 1, Drink 2
Day 5-6 Drink: Morning Glory, Drink 3, Drink 4

Morning Glory (Daily Shake)

3 cups of greens
2 cups of seeds (sprouted)
2 cups of sprouts
½ apple
½ avocado
2 tbl sea vegetable (**Chlorella, Dulse, Kelp, Nori** (aka laver), **Spirulina, Wakame)**
Himalayan salt (to taste)
Cayenne pepper
5 ½ cups of water

Drink as much as you like of the morning glory.

Drink 1:
Drink 16 oz. once a day.
1 lemon
½ Lime
Cayenne pepper to taste
16 0z of spring water (alkaline is better)

Drink 2:
 2 Apples
3 celery stalk
1 cucumber
1 ½ tsp ginger
½ lemon with peel
1 lime with peel
3 cups of spinach
1 bunch of parsley
5 ½ cups of water

This is a lot of ingredients. It may be too thick for you to drink. I recommend placing half the ingredients in the blender fill with spring water (or alkaline) and blend. Pour into a separate container and repeat with the remainder of the ingredients. Mix both containers well and drink for 3 days.

Drink 3:
3 cups of spinach
1 apple
½ cup of blueberries
4 cups of water (spring or alkaline)

Drink 4:
Pure Organic cranberry juice from health store. Or make your own
        Drink once a day

During the 5 day kidney cleanse, you are to drink shakes only. If you're not able to go without eating, eat a salad or veggie snacks. (Celery, cucumbers) It doesn't matter how much salad you eat because all of them are raw.

Day 7-8

Spirit: (minimum)

	Prayer	once daily
	Mediation	times a day

Skin

	Brushing	once daily
	Water	Drink ½ your body weight in ounces
	Sweat	Daily

Lungs

	Deep breathing	all day
	Breathing Exercise	3 times a day

Preparation for Liver cleanse:

Consume 1 quart of organic unsweetened apple juice once a day for 3 days. Make sure the last of the apple juice is consumed by 2pm on the 9th day.

Homemade Apple smoothie:

Blend 3 organic apples to a quart of water.

You may eat all the recipes in the book. You can try others.

Instructions

Liver & Colon Cleanse (Start day 9)

Day 9

Mix in a jar and place in the refrigerator

Jar 1
4 tbsp. Epson salt
3 cups of water

Jar 2
½ cup of Olive oil
½ cup grapefruit or lemon juice
10 to 20 drops black walnut hull tincture (health store)

2:00 P.M. Do not eat or drink after 2 o'clock. If you break this rule you could feel sick later.

Mix your epsom salt and water and place in the refrigerator.

6:00 PM. Drink ¾ cup for the epsom salt mixture. You may rinse your mouth with water

Get the olive oil and grapefruit out to warm up.

8:00 P.M. Repeat by drinking another ¾ cup of Epsom salts.

You haven't eaten since two o'clock, but you won't feel hungry.

Get your bedtime chores done. The timing is critical for success.

9:45 P.M. Pour ½ cup olive oil (for best results into the pint jar.) Squeeze the grapefruit or lemon by hand into the measuring cup. Remove pulp with fork. You should have at least ½ cup. Add this to the olive oil. Also, add Black Walnut Hull Tincture.

You visit the bathroom one or more times, even if it makes you late for your ten o'clock drink. Don't be more than 15 minutes late. You will get fewer stones.

10:00 P.M. Drink the potion you have mixed. Drinking through a large plastic straw helps it go down easier. You may use salad dressing, syrup, or straight sweetener to chase it down between sips. Take it to your bedside if you wish. Get it down within five minutes (15 minutes for very elderly or weak persons). If you had difficulty getting stones out in the past add ½ tsp. citric acid to the potion.

Lie down immediately. You might fail to get stones out if you don't. The sooner you lie down the more stones you will get out. Be ready for bed ahead of time. Don't clean up the kitchen. As soon as the drink is down walk to your bed and lie down flat on your back with your head up high on the pillow. Try to think about what is happening in the liver. Try to keep perfectly still for at least 20 minutes. You may feel a train of stones traveling along the bile ducts like marbles. There is no pain because the bile duct valves are open (thank you Epsom salts!). Go to sleep, you may fail to get stones out if you don't. Sleep on your side.

Day 10

Spirit: (minimum)

Prayer	1 once daily
Mediation	3 times a day

Skin

Brushing	1 once daily
Water	Drink ½ of your body weight in ounces daily
Sweat	Daily

Lungs

Deep breathing	all day
Breathing Exercise	3 times a day

Next morning. Upon awakening take your third dose of Epsom salts. If you have indigestion or nausea wait until it is gone before drinking the Epsom salts. You may go back to bed. Don't take this potion before 6:00 am.

2 Hours Later. Take your fourth (the last) dose of Epsom salts. You may go back to bed again.

After 2 More Hours you may eat. Start with fruit juice. Half an hour later eat fruit. One hour later you may eat regular food but keep it light. During the day take the parasite-killing herbs and zap. By dinner you should feel recovered.

Additional Recipes

Oatmeal Raisin Cookies

2 cup of oatmeal

¼ cup raisins

4 dates

1 tsp cinnamon

¼ cup of Costa Rica sugar

½ tsp vanilla extract

Mix the ingredients together. Spoon out mixture and form on a paraflexx sheet. Place in the dehydrator for 5 hours.

If you don't have a dehydrator form balls and enjoy!

BROWNIES
1 cup Cashews
1 cup raw almonds
2 ½ pitted dates (soak)
¾ cup cacao powder
2 tbsp. cacao nibs
Pinch of salt
Mix all ingredients. Pour in a Pyrex pan. Sit for 1 hour and serve.

Mojito

Ingredients:
1 cup Grapes
½ cup of mint
½ cup of spinach
½ cup of coconut water
1 tablespoon of lime juice
2 tsp chia seeds

Lemonade Smoothie

> 1 cup water
> 1 Lemon (peeled)
> ⅓ Blueberries
> ½ stalk celery

Superfoods Salad

Mixed Greens, Sprouted Sunflower Seeds, Flaxseeds, Avocado, Cucumber, Red, orange and yellow sweet pepper

Add as much as you like

Mock Chicken Curry Salad

½ cup almonds (soaked)

½ cup Cashews (soaked)

2 tbsp. celery

2 tsp diced onions

1 tsp Relish or Kalamata Olive

1 tsp Poultry Seasoning

1 tsp marjoram

¼ tsp dill

½ tsp lemon juice

½ tsp apple cider vinegar

Curried avocado mayo (½ avocado, 1 tsp curried ½ tbsp. water)

3 Leaves Romaine Lettuce

Blend cashews and almonds to a creamy slightly crunchy

Mix all the ingredients together adding mayo last. Everyone likes different taste, so add or subtract to your liking. Serve on Romaine Lettuce.

References:

(Thank all of you for your knowledge)

Clark, H. (2007). *The cure and prevention of all cancers.* Chula Vista, CA: New Century Press.

Global Healing Center; by Dr. Edward Group DC, NP, DACBN, DCBCN, DABFM Published on October 30, 2012, Last Updated on August 8, 2014

Global Healing Center ;by Dr. Edward Group DC, NP, DACBN, DCBCN, DABFM Published on February 11, 2015, Last Updated on February 13, 2015

Morning Glory daily shake was inspired by "Living Foods Institute"

www.ingramcontent.com/pod-product-compliance
Lightning Source LLC
Chambersburg PA
CBHW072017280526
45788CB00005B/2079